Diabetes: Powerful Superfoods that Drastically Lower Your Blood Sugar Level

by Diabetic Mastery

Table of Contents

Free Gift

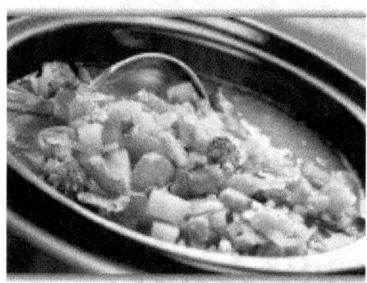

Click Here!!!!!!

As a "Thank You" for downloading this book I want to offer you **"*Diabetic Mastery Slow Cooker Recipes"*** eBook as well as full access to Diabetic Mastery's reading list. Once you join this email list you will receive not only this free eBook instantly but you also receive some of the most valuable information in this topic ranging from book, newsletters, videos, article, and much more!!!!. Once again thank you downloading and we hope you enjoy!!!!!!!

Introduction

High blood sugar level simply refers to a health situation where the level of sugar glucose in the blood becomes elevated. It is otherwise known as hyperglycemia. High blood sugar often exists in people with issues of diabetes mellitus. High blood sugar often leads to the spillage of glucose into the urine thereby giving the urine a sugary taste.

The real meaning of the term diabetes mellitus is sweet urine. Diabetes mellitus is not the only known cause of high blood sugar cases. High blood sugar can also be caused by the consumption of much sugary foods and fruits than the body needs. Some of these other causes of diabetes mellitus include: the presence of any infection, an injury, post surgery stress and other illnesses.

High blood sugar may not produce any symptoms at all, but sometimes, certain symptoms are associated with this condition. When there are symptoms, the most common symptoms may include: frequent urination, thirst, dry mouth, blurry vision, urinating during the night, dry mouth, fatigue, weight loss, drowsiness, and increased hunger pangs.

An increased level of blood sugar may be an indication that one is at an increased risk of heart attack. The risk of dying from heart attacks has been found to increase in people with increased blood sugar level.

The opposite of high blood sugar is low blood sugar which is also known as hypoglycemia. There are several foods that contribute to the increase in blood sugar levels. Your body also uses some chemicals to create more glucose in the liver and the muscles. The human blood is responsible for carrying the blood sugar to all cells in the human body. To take glucose to all body cells as sources of energy, the cells need the help of insulin. Insulin is a hormone produced by the pancreas

The pancreas in responsible for the release of insulin into the human blood, depending on the blood sugar levels. Insulin is quite useful in transporting digested foods into the cells. The body can stop the production of insulin as can be seen in type 1 diabetes, the insulin can equally stop working properly as can be seen in type 2 diabetes. In people with diabetes, glucose fails to go into the cells in sufficient amount, which makes it get lodged in the blood causing an increase in the blood sugar levels.

The blood glucose meter can be used to measure the blood sugar levels. This meter is also known as glucometer. The test for blood sugar level is simple, just place a tiny drop of blood from the forearm or finger into the test strip and insert the strip into the glucometer. The blood sugar level is digitally displayed within seconds.

The blood glucose levels vary widely all through the day and night in diabetic patients. Naturally, the blood glucose levels range between 30 and 130 mg/dL before a meal and below 180 mg/dL between 1 and 2 hours after a meal.

People with diabetes often try to keep their blood sugar levels under control between the within the range of 80-150 mg/dL before meals. Health practitioners and educators help patients determine their highest range of blood sugar control.

When the level of blood sugar stay high for a very long time, like for a couple of hours, more serious problems like dehydration and other such complications can arise. Moreover, even mild cases of hyperglycemia when poorly treated or unrecognized for a number of years can lead to the damage of multiple tissues in the brain, kidney, and arteries.

When hyperglycemia is associated with cases of ketones in the urine, it calls for urgent medical attention to forestall the deterioration of the problem. When the level of blood sugar rises and stay long for several days or weeks, diabetes may be the major cause and must be given adequate treatment immediately.

There are several high blood sugar level fluctuations in diabetic patients on a daily basis. It is very important to control the level of blood sugar through exercises, diets, or prescribed medication, with the aim of knowing the symptoms of high blood sugar levels, and to seek urgent medical attention whenever it becomes necessary.

Causes of Increase in Blood Sugar levels

A number of things can be responsible for increased in blood sugar level, but some of these causes are more prevalent than the others. Diabetes mellitus has been identified by experts as one of the major causes of high blood sugar levels. High blood sugar in people with diabetes can be caused by a number of factors such as:

Carbohydrates

Eating food that contains lots of carbohydrates, which is a form of sugar can lead to increased blood sugar levels in people with diabetes.

The body of diabetic patient lacks the ability to process high level of carbohydrates with the speed required for them to be converted into energy. In diabetic patients, blood sugar can rise to very high levels within some seconds after a meal.

Insulin control

- The absence of adequate insulin action can lead to high sugar levels. The insulin level in the human body can be controlled by injection of insulin or taking medications that regulate the pancreas ability to produce insulin.

- It is important for diabetic patients to control their blood sugar levels using a combination of dietary discretion, physical activities and taking medications. When there is no balance between food, exercises and insulin levels, the blood sugar level rises automatically.

Stress

- Your physical emotions can play very vital role in causing blood sugar levels to rise, but this should never be an excuse for not controlling your diabetes.

Inadequate exercises

- Daily exercise is one of the most critical factors when it comes to the regulation of blood sugar levels.

Diseases

- When there is any ailment in the body of an individual, the blood sugar levels tend to rise at a very high rate over several hours.

Other medications

- Certain medications, especially steroidal drugs can have a very high effect on the blood sugar levels.

Symptoms of High Blood Sugar Levels

High blood sugar level on its own is a symptom of diabetes mellitus. However, a diabetes mellitus patient may not experience any kind of symptoms at all.

Common symptoms of diabetes mellitus include:

- Thirst
- Dry mouth
- Frequent urination
- Urinating during the night
- Dry, itchy skin
- Blurry vision
- Fatigue and drowsiness
- Weight loss
- Increased appetite

However, other symptoms may develop if diabetes persist for several hours and results in dehydration. Some of these symptoms that come with dehydration in prolonged cases of high blood sugar include:

- Dizziness when standing

- Difficulty with breathing
- Increased confusion and drowsiness
- Unconsciousness or coma

When left untreated for too long, high blood sugar level scan lead to a case known as ketoacidosis or diabetic coma. This case arise due to the fact that the body of a person with high blood sugar level has insufficient insulin to handle the processing of glucose into fuel, so the body breaks down fats and use it as energy.

When the body breaks down fats, ketones are formed as by-products. Some ketones are gotten rid of via the urine, but not all the ketones. Ketones remain in the blood until the patient is rehydrated and insulin action fully restored. The presence of ketones in the blood can lead to cases such as headache, fatigue, vomiting, nausea, etc.

Ketoacidosis is a life-threatening condition that requires immediate treatment. The symptoms of this condition include:

- Nausea and vomiting
- Shortness of breath
- Breath that smells fruity

- Stomach pain
- Dry mouth

When to seek medical attention

If hyperglycemia persists for more than two days, or if there are ketones in the urine, you should do well to call in your doctor for medical help.

People suffering from diabetes are advised to test their blood sugar levels about four times daily: before meals and before bedtime. You can equally follow the advice by your medical expert for individual diabetes care plans. Anytime the blood sugar levels rises above 250mg/dL, the urine should be checked for the presence of ketones.

When the blood sugar levels remain high despite having followed the right diabetic diet and care plan, call the diabetic health educator, nurse, or physician for diet adjustment.

If any of the following symptoms develop, seek medical attention

- Confusion

- Sleepiness

- Vomiting

- Dehydration

- Shortness of breath

- The presence of ketones in the urine

- Glucose readings higher than 300 mg/dL

- Blood sugar levels that stay 160 mg/dL for longer than one week

All cases of ketoacidosis or diabetic coma is a very serious medical emergency and must be treated as such by calling 911 to provide you with emergency transportation to a nearby hospital or any other medical emergency center.

Care, treatments and prevention for high Blood sugar

To care for your blood sugar levels adequately, you must know certain important facts about blood sugar levels. Below are certain questions you need to ask your doctor to enable you understand everything you need to know about your blood sugar levels.

- How you can recognize your blood sugar levels

- How to treat a high blood sugar level when it develops in you, a friend, co worker or family member

- How you can prevent your blood sugar level from becoming too high

- How to get in touch with the medical staff during an emergency situation

- The emergency supplies you need to treat high blood sugar

- Additional educational materials you should always carry as regards properly handling of high blood sugar levels.

Self-Care at Home

Check your blood sugar levels using a blood glucose meter. If the blood sugar level is higher than what it should be, without any trace of the common symptoms of high blood sugar levels, continue to administer routine care like the following:

- Taking all diabetic drugs according to medical schedules and recommendations

- Eating meals regularly

- Drinking sugar-free and caffeine-free liquids always

- Taking your blood sugar readings every four hours until such a time when your blood sugar levels return to normal

- Check our urine for the presence of ketones and make sure you put down the readings you get. Follow the sick day rules outlined in your diabetes care plan by your doctor until no trace of ketones can be found in your urine.

How to lower blood sugar levels

There are certain tested and trusted strategies to help you lower your blood sugar levels, and some of these strategies include:

Exercise

One of the simplest ways to lower your blood sugar levels is through exercises. But when your blood sugar levels get higher than 240 mg/dL, first check for ketones in your urine.

If there are traces of ketones, do not embark on any exercises. The reason you should abstain from exercise when there are ketones in your blood is because exercising will even make your sugar levels to rise even higher.

Talk to your doctor about the safest and easiest ways to lower your blood glucose levels in this kind of situation.

Diet

work with a diabetes health educator or registered dietitian to come up with a workable diet plan to help you manage diabetes.

Medication

If following the recommended diets and exercise fail to regulate your blood sugar levels, the doctor may have to adjust the timing, amount, or type of insulin or medications for you.

Treating High Blood Sugar

Treating high blood sugar may not be too easy, but it is quite possible. There are different ways you can go about treating your high blood sugar. The following are some very effective treatments you can adopt for managing your blood sugar levels whenever there is a rise.

Change of medication

High blood sugar may be a sign that there is an urgent need for a change in medication in a diabetic patient. To change medication or the way it is administered, there may be an addition to the quantity of insulin given, or there may be a switch from any medications to injected medications.

Other diseases

If an illness is responsible for the rise in the blood sugar levels, the illness should be diagnosed and treated without any delays. Illnesses and infections may have to be treated in the hospital, where health practitioners can adjust their plan of care.

Other medications

There are a number of medications you can use for the control of blood sugar levels and type 2 diabetes. Insulin is also recommended, especially for people with diabetes whether type 1 or type 2.

Follow-up techniques for treating diabetes

Diabetic patients are advised to get a hemoglobin A1c test performed once in three months. Similar to a report card, this test provides feedback about the total sugar levels within the three months period.

Diabetic patients ought to have a hemoglobin A1c level below 7% at each clinical visit. Most cases where the hemoglobin A1c levels are above the 7% benchmark are as a result of the patient's failure to:

- Take the prescribed medications
- Follow the proper diet plans
- Closely Monitor the blood glucose
- failure to embark of proper exercises or
- lack of good judgment and proper motivation regarding the recommended high blood sugar management plans.

Preventive techniques for high blood sugar

- Get all the necessary knowledge on proper management of high blood sugar.
- Work with a certified diabetes expert. This educator should have a CDE certification and may be a worker in either a hospital or a diabetic education center.
- Check your blood sugar as recommended by your doctor, nurse or CDE.

- Know the common symptoms of high blood sugar before the condition spirals of control.
- Follow a diabetes diet plan and make adjustments to the plan as needed.

Take diabetic medications as recommended by your medical practitioner.

Why Blood Sugar Rises

Several factors have been linked with the increase in blood sugar levels. Apart from diseases like diabetes, choice of foods and certain lifestyles are some other major causes of high blood sugar levels. Below are some of the major causes of rise in blood sugar levels.

Sugar-free foods

Most foods that claim to be sugar-free play a big role in increasing your blood sugar levels. The reason for this can be linked to the fact that many of these foods contain carbohydrates in the form of fats, starches, and fiber.

Some sugar alcohols such as xylitol and sorbitol add the necessary sweetness to these sugar-free foods, but these sugar alcohols contain high amounts of associated carbohydrates to cause a rise in your blood sugar levels.

Foods that contain very high carbohydrates have the ability to cause your blood sugar levels to rise to very high levels, and may eventually cause organ damage in diabetic patients.

Caffeine

There are several ways blood sugar can be affected and result in complications in the control of sugar levels in diabetic patients. Each individual has a different way of reacting to various items that can influence the blood sugar levels.

People with diabetes should always examine some food items to find out the effect they may have on their blood sugar levels. Blood sugar levels may increase after taking coffee, black tea, and some energy drinks because they contain caffeine.

There are several other items that can affect your blood sugar levels and methods you can use to determine the effect of different compounds on your blood sugar levels.

Chinese Foods

Most Chinese foods have been found to be very high in fats. Foods that contain high amounts of fats can cause your blood sugar to stay high for a very long time.

French fries, pizza, and most of the fried foods you find in Chinese restaurants contain very high amounts of both carbohydrates and fats, and are therefore not good for you.

Checking your blood sugar levels two hours after the intake of such foods will enable you know how they affect your blood sugar levels.

Cold

A bad cold causes dehydration, and dehydration can cause a rise in your blood sugar levels. If you are sick, vomiting and diarrhea that lasts longer than two hours or illnesses that linger for days can raise your blood sugar levels, especially when there is dehydration.

It is important stay as hydrated as possible when you are sick as a way of fighting high blood sugar levels. The blood sugar levels in the body are known to rise as your body tries to fight off some rampaging diseases.

Medications like antibiotics and certain decongestants can change your blood sugar levels. Check your blood sugar levels regularly, especially when you are sick to know how your body is reacting to certain disease conditions and treatments.

Stress

Stress, especially job stress have been found to contribute to the rise in blood sugar levels. Though this is more prevalent in people with type 2 diabetes, practicing some relaxation techniques with deep breathing and exercises will help you reduce your stress levels. Reducing your stress levels will help you regulate your blood sugar swings.

Bagels

To some people, bagel is better than the regular bread, but in reality, bagels are only better when it comes to causing an increase in your blood sugar levels. This is because bagels are loaded with carbohydrates and calories.

If you must have a bagel at all, make sure you choose a mini bagel. You can discuss with your dietician or health practitioner for healthier alternatives.

Sports Drinks

Sports drinks are designed to help people replenish lost fluids fast, but many of these sports drinks come with a very large amount of sugars.

Pure table water is always a better alternative, especially when you are on a workout that lasts less than an hour. Though sports drinks are more appropriate for more intense workouts, but it is important to consult your doctor for medical advice on which sports drink you should go for.

Dried Fruits

Though fruits are healthy choices for maintaining a overall well being, people with diabetes should abstain from dried fruits as they contain very large amounts of carbohydrates.

Each small serving of dried fruits comes with loads of carbohydrates which is not healthy. Researches have shown that two tablespoons of cranberries, dried raisins, or cherries contain the same amount of carbohydrates as a piece of fresh fruit. Eating a handful of dried fruits may cause an unwanted spike in your blood sugar levels.

Steroids and water pills

Steroids, which are mostly used for treating cases like rashes, asthma, arthritis, and several other medical conditions can cause a rise in blood sugar levels.

Corticosteroids like prednisone can cause diabetes in healthy individuals. Diuretics may cause a rise in blood sugar levels, while antidepressants may either raise or lower your blood sugar levels.

If you are diabetic and need any of these medications, make sure you monitor your blood sugar levels regularly to see the effects of these medications on you.

Cold Medicines

Cold medicines often contain pseudoephredine or phenylphrine as decongestants; they may also contain sugar or alcohol. These components can cause a rise in your blood sugar levels.

Antihistamines don't cause any kind of problems with your blood sugar levels. If you purchase your cold medicines over the counter, make sure you ask your pharmacist about the possible effects of the medicines on your blood sugar levels.

Rollercoaster Effects on Blood Sugar

Apart from the above mentioned causes of increase in blood sugar levels, there are some other factors that have been identified to have rollercoaster effects on your blood sugar. Below are some of the factors that may have rollercoaster effects on your blood sugar levels.

Exercises

It is a known fact that physical exercises can help improve your overall health and well being. Even in people with diabetes, exercises can still help them maintain optimum health.

But, it is important to note that when people with diabetes embark on endurance or intense type of exercises, their blood sugar levels may rise and then fall.

People suffering from diabetes should always check their blood sugar levels before, during and after intense physical exercises to make sure their blood sugar levels do not rise too high.

Adequate monitoring of your blood sugar levels coupled with the right treatments, can help you regulate the rollercoaster effects of exercises on your blood sugar levels.

Alcohol

When people with diabetes drink alcohol, the same rollercoaster effects exercises have on your blood sugar levels can equally occur. When you take alcohol, your blood sugar levels rises to a very high level before falling.

When they fall, they remain low for as long as 12 hours. This rollercoaster effect of alcohol on your blood sugar can be adequately controlled when you eat while you drink.

Alcohol drinks can also come with loads of carbohydrates. Experts opine that women should take only one alcoholic beverage per day, while men are advised to take about two and not more daily.

Heat

Being too hot makes the control of your blood sugar levels quite difficult. Going in and out of a room with an air conditioner can have a rollercoaster effect on your blood sugar levels.

Staying in an air-conditioned room during a hot day can help you keep your blood sugar levels normal. Drinking lots of water to avoid being dehydrated is another way you can prevent a rise in your blood sugar levels on a hot day.

It is important to keep all diabetes medications, glucose meter and test strips under room temperature as heats in cars and from windowsills can affect them negatively.

Female Hormones

Hormone changes is yet another cause of change in blood sugar levels. During menstrual circles and menopause in women, the changes that occur in female hormones make the blood sugar levels to fluctuate.

Constant monitoring of blood sugar levels can help people with diabetes manage their blood sugar level changes that occur as a result of hormonal changes. Discuss hormone replacement therapy with your doctor and how these hormones can affect your blood sugar changes.

How bad is sugar for you?

If you are an incurable alcoholic with a sweet tooth and a serious case of diabetes, you may not have to give up these sugary items forever. The important thing is for you understand the fact that sugar will cause a rise in your blood sugar levels, faster than any other carbohydrate can.

The total amount of carbohydrate contained in your food is another very important factor you must always consider too. Consequently, if people with diabetes can control a serving size and keep it small, they can enjoy all the foods they love the most so long as they take the amount of carbohydrates and calories contained in these foods into consideration.

Taking the amount of carbohydrates and calories in your foods into consideration will enable you ensure they don't exceed their usual dietary intakes. This simply means that a small serving of sweets should naturally offset foods that contain no sweets at all.

What should you know about glycemic index?

The glycemic index of any food is a measure of how an individual's blood sugar levels is raised by that particular food. Knowing your total daily consumption of carbohydrate is one way you can manage your blood sugar levels.

As a result, eating whole grains and beans with lower glycemic index than pasta or white bread can help keep your blood sugar levels low. So if you need to take a very small amount of high glycemic index foods like a small piece of pie, it will be advisable you make the rest of your total carbohydrate intake for the day from low glycemic index foods.

Dangers of High Blood Sugar

It is a well known fact that high blood sugar causes a number of health-related complications, but the question is, have you ever wondered why this condition is injurious to your health and what dangers are associated with it?

There are no obvious symptoms of diabetes, but sometimes, you can hear people say high blood sugar is good for them. But, experts in the health industry will always tell you that there is no such thing as your blood sugar being a little bit high or having a touch of diabetes.

Blood sugar coats red blood cells and helps make them stiff. These sticky hemoglobin interfere with the proper circulation of the blood, which leads to a buildup of cholesterol on the inside of your blood vessels.

It can take a couple of years before the damage this condition causes to your body can become very noticeable.

The parts of your body that are most susceptible to this condition include: your kidneys, your eyes, and your feet. Problems are usually first noticed in these parts of the body.

Controlling your blood sugar levels has been linked to very high success rate when it comes to the control of long-term complications that may arise from diabetes. Some of these long-term diabetes complications include:

- Stroke
- Heart attacks
- Nerve damage in your hands and feet that can cause you pain, numbness and tingling sensations
- Eye problems that can result in complications with your eyesight or blindness.
- Kidney failures and other kidney problems
- Gum disease and tooth loss

Some of these damages to the body may start way before diabetes set in a stage known as the prediabetes stage. This prediabetes stage is a condition in which your blood sugar rises higher than the normal levels, but not high enough to be considered a diabetic case.

According to researches, if you have prediabetes, your risk of developing type 2 diabetes reduces by almost 60% through change in lifestyle. Some of these changes include increasing your physical activity and modest weight loss.

Ultimately, diabetes is a very chronic disease that is capable of affecting several aspects of your health and overall well being. It is important that you always take cases involving high blood sugar very seriously. Regular follow-up care may be helpful for proper management of the disease and will go a long way to enable you live a more active healthier life.

Foods that increase your blood sugar levels

Candy

High-sugar foods such as candy, syrup, cookies and soda lack nutritional values, but a more serious effect of these low-quality carbohydrates is that they can cause very dramatic spike in your blood sugar levels and can contribute immensely to your weight gains.

Both of these negative effects of these high-sugar foods can make diabetes cases worse. Get yourself accustomed to eating high-quality carbohydrates like fresh fruits.

Apples, berries, grapes, oranges and pears all have very juicy sweet flavors and contain a lot of fibers, which are beneficial in slowing the absorption of glucose, making them much better and healthier choices for blood sugar control.

Whenever you have to snack on foods like string cheese, low-fat yogurt, a handful of nuts, to further reduce the impact they have on your blood sugar levels.

Fruit Juice

While whole fruits are very healthy, fiber-rich carbohydrate options for diabetes patients, the same cannot exactly be said about fruit juice.

Though fruit juice offers more nutritional value than soda and all other sugary drinks, but fruit juices-even when they are 100% natural are made up of fruit sugar, and as a result cause a very sharp spike in blood sugar.

Skipping that glass of fruit juice you love so much and opting for a more fiber-rich whole fruit alternative may be all you need to maintain a very healthy blood sugar levels.

Going for this healthier alternative will equally help you get filled up on fewer calories, which aids weight loss. For a more refreshing and healthy drink alternative, go for zero calorie plain or naturally-flavored seltzer with some wedge of lime or lemon.

Raisins

Eating raisins have been found to be a healthier better option than snacking on cookies, but it will still raise your sugar levels. Eating every other dried fruit have the same effects on your sugar levels.

The reason for this is because during dehydration process, natural sugars from fruits become more concentrated, thereby causing a very unhealthy rise in your blood sugar levels when they get absorbed rapidly into your body.

This is one more reason to stick with whole, fresh fruit options such as cantaloupe, grapefruits, strawberries and peaches.

Fried Foods

Overdoing it on your passion for greasy fries can do a lot of damage to your blood sugar levels apart from the obvious weight gain effects that accompany such choice of foods.

Foods like French fries as mentioned earlier, potato chips, and doughnuts are very bad food choices because they are made from very unhealthy carb-heavy, starchy ingredients, which can cause a high increase in your blood sugar levels. Fried foods when being prepared soak up several tons of oil, which adds lots of extra calories to these fried foods. Some fried foods like fried chicken and fried appetizers are coated in breading and this increases their calorie more.

Pancakes and syrups

One of the worst breakfast choices for someone suffering from diabetes is a plate of pancakes with syrup. Most pancakes are jumbo sized and are made from junky white flours. So taking about three large pancakes can be the equivalent of taking about seven slices of white bread.

the toppings even make matters worse. Butter is loaded with saturated fats that clog the arteries. A typical half-cup pour of gooey pancake syrup can add about 16 straight teaspoons of sugar to your breakfast.

This dangerous combination of starch and sugar will no doubt send your blood sugar levels spiraling to the high heavens, not to mention their negative effects on your weight.

Next time you visit a diner, pay no attention to the pancakes. You can order some low-carb, protein-rich egg white omelet laced with some vegetables.

White Bread

All refined starches such as: white bread, white pasta, white rice, and anything produced from white flour behave like sugar the moment the body begins to digest them.

Therefore, just like you avoid sugar, all refined starches interfere with blood sugar control and should be kept at a safe distance by those suffering from diabetes.

Whole grains are better options because they are richer in fiber and generally cause a slower steadier rise in the blood sugar levels.

Instead of going for white bread or bagel for breakfast, you should choose something like a whole grain English Muffin topped with a slice of reduced-fat cheese or scrambled egg for protein.

At lunch and dinner, replace the white carb foods with healthier whole grains like brown rice, quinoa, barley, as well as whole wheat bread to reduce their effects on your blood sugar levels.

Whole Milk

For people with diabetes, a diet with very high saturated fat content can make your insulin resistance worse. Keep whole milk out of your fridge and go for skim milk instead.

Make sure you avoid all dairy products like full-fat yogurt, cream, cream and regular cheese. Choose their reduced fat alternatives whenever you need to take them.

Snacks and Pastries

It is a very common knowledge that all bakes and packaged foods are loaded with sodium, sugar, junky white flours and lots of preservatives.

The dangerous combination of sugar and refined flour raises your blood sugar levels and promotes the inflammation of some body organs, which inhibits the proper functioning of insulin in your body.

25 super foods that lower your blood sugar levels

There are several tips and pieces of advice from health experts to help people with diabetes manage their blood sugar levels. The most effective of these tips has to do with foods that help lower your blood sugar levels. These foods that help lower your blood sugar level may not be very effective if you do not know how best to incorporate them into your daily diet.

Researches have shown that the best foods for diabetes remain those unprocessed foods like fruits and vegetables. Adding these foods that have extra health benefits will not only add more nutritional values to your diet, but will go a long way to help meet your health needs like lowering your blood sugar levels and preventing all diseases associated with diabetes such as heart attacks.

Most of these super foods are able to control your blood sugar levels as a result of their abilities to lower the digestion rates. Lowering the rate at which foods are digested in your body ensure the slow and steady release of blood sugar into your body. Below are the top 25 foods that can help lower your blood sugar levels, why they are super foods and how to incorporate them into your diet.

Beans

Beans are known to be very nutritious low-fat sources of good protein, but there are more things that make them super foods. Beans are very high in fiber, which means they are quite good at slowing down the rate at which foods are digested. Beans can be taken alone or mixed with other low-fat grains and legumes.

Fish

High blood sugar can put your heart at a very great risk, so you will want to do whatever possible to make sure your heart is always protected. Choosing healthy lean protein for your diet is one way you can achieve this. Fish is one of those food sources that add nothing to your blood sugar levels, but instead brings the all important omega-3 fatty acids to the table to make sure your heart is kept safe from the rampaging sugars from sugary food sources. Fish can be part of every meal as a way of beefing up the nutrient level of your food.

Carrots

Carrots are some great foods you can easily incorporate into your diet to keep your blood sugar low. Carrots whether cooked or raw delivers the required amount of fiber to give you a feeling of fullness and help slow the digestion process.

Carrots can be chopped and added as dressings for your salad and some other foods like rice. It can equally be eaten as dessert. Studies have shown that when eaten raw, carrots deliver more fibers and other nutrients to your body.

Apples

Whoever said one apple a day keeps the doctor away couldn't have been closer to the truth. Apples contain the right amount of vitamins and minerals needed by the body to carry out all metabolitic processes.

Making apple a part of your diet will ensure you reduce your intake of sugary and starchy foods that may be harmful to your health and raise your blood sugar levels. Apples can be taken as meal replacements or before meals to minimize the quantity of foods you need to consume.

Apples have also been found to be very healthy options for desserts due to their health benefits and the fact that they help reduce your blood sugar levels.

Oats

For several decades, oats have continued to provide the needed health benefits due to their ability to help diabetes patients manage the condition. People who take oats are equally known to take oats as a preventive measure against diabetes.

Oats are equally very beneficial when it comes to regulating the blood sugar levels in your body. Oats are able to keep your blood sugar levels low for several hours after your oat meals.

Oats also provide your body with good amount of fiber which helps lower the rates at which your body digests foods. Oats are equally helpful in the management of conditions like high cholesterol and high blood pressure.

These qualities make oat an overall healthy foods that help you stay in top health all through the day. Oats can be taken during breakfast to help you energy levels remain stable and your sugar levels low all through the day.

Peas

Oats are known to come with very low amount of calories, which makes them ideal to be incorporated into any kind of meat-based meal as a side dish. They equally contain the right amount of potassium and are high in fiber content.

Apart from keeping your blood sugar levels in check, peas are good sources of vitamin C and proteins for your overall health and wellbeing. They can be taken with any meal at any time of the day as a side dish and still deliver their full nutritional benefits.

Peas and carrots make a very great side dish when mixed together. They are not just delicious when combined, but helps your goal of keeping your blood sugar levels low alive.

Broccoli

Broccoli is known to be one super food that can come with lots of health benefits. It is an anti-inflammatory food, helps prevent cancer, and does so much more to keep you in the best health conditions.

This low glycemic food ensures your blood sugar levels are kept as low as possible. Broccoli makes a great side dish because of its ability to provide your body with lots of fiber, protein, vitamins and minerals.

You can get a nice nutritional spread from just one serving of broccoli. Broccoli serves as a great side dish during breakfast and super.

Cabbage

The fact that cabbage contains very low fat and comes with very low calories makes it a great dietary super food.

Cabbage is known to be quite versatile due to its ability to find its way into several great dishes and recipes. It serves a very good side dish when steamed until it gets very soft. It is known to provide texture, flavor and nutrition to foods. The dose of vitamin C it contains makes it helpful for strengthening your immune system.

Kale

Kale is a very legal superfood so you can enjoy it whenever and however you want without any worries that it will raise your blood sugar levels. Kale is known to provide your body with essential vitamins like C and A.

It is equally a very good source of fiber, which helps lower the rate your body digests foods. It provides your body with as much potassium as banana and serves as a good source of iron.

Its fat and calorie contents are quite low as well. Kale is a great addition to your regular intake of fruits and vegetables. It can be taken before, during or after meals.

Tomatoes

Tomatoes are very popular for their ability to help prevent and control diseases like cancer and heart attacks. Their low glycemic index makes them useful in a large number of ways.

The best way to eat tomatoes is perhaps to make a sauce out of them because their nutritional factor gets compounded after they have been cooked. They can be eaten raw as a salad and can even be blended as to produce tomato juice.

They are quite good for maintaining a low blood sugar level due to their low glycemic index. Eating them regularly is one way of taking care of the overall health needs of your body.

Cauliflower

When it comes to foods that do not spike up your blood sugar levels, cauliflower plays a very important part. The previously mentioned kale and cabbage falls into this category as well.

These vegetables are always in the news as superfoods due to their anti-cancer and anti-heart diseases effects.

Their unique blend of phytonutrients is well received by the body, and eating them regularly does not only help maintain a low blood sugar levels as they have very low glycemic index but goes a long way to maintain your overall good health.

You can rotate your intake of these great vegetables to make sure you don't eat the same vegetable daily. Cauliflower can be used to make faux-tatoes as well as pizza crust.

Whole Wheat Bread

Whole wheat breads have continued to gain more popularity in recent years due to the fact that white breads have been linked to a number of health problems. Apart from the fact that the body is able to process whole wheat bread more efficiently than it processes white bread.

Whole wheat bread comes with a much lower glycemic index than white bread, which means they are quite beneficial to keeping your blood sugar levels low. Whole wheat bread can be eaten with your low-fat low-sugar beverages during breakfast.

Mushrooms

Certain species of mushrooms are known to provide the body with a number of health benefits. Apart from the great flavor and nutritional values these edible mushrooms add to your meals, the fact that they help keep your blood sugar levels low as each of them comes with a very low glycemic index makes them some of the most delicious and nutritious superfoods. You can easily incorporate mushrooms into your meals as spices in soups and stews.

Quinoa

The recent popularity this food is enjoying in the food and nutrition market is not unconnected to the fact that it has been found to be both gluten-free and grain-free. The fact that this superfood comes with very low sugar content makes it suitable for keeping blood sugar levels at an all time low. Apart from the health benefits of quinoa, it comes with loads of fiber, protein, and a very nice mix of both vitamins and minerals.

Cherries

When it comes to foods that do not spike up your blood sugar levels, cherries are one of such superfoods that should easily come to mind. Cherries can be sour or sweet, but one thing you can always be sure of is the fact that they provide you with important vitamins like vitamin A and vitamin C. They are equally very low in fat and calorie content. With their low glycemic index, they do not spike up your blood glucose levels.

Coconut

When eaten sparingly, coconut can be a good source of sweetness to your meals without causing any harm to your blood sugar levels. Coconut comes with high fat content. It can be used to flavor a wide variety of dishes using different parts of it like the water, the milk, the flour, as well as the flesh.

Peaches

When they are in season, peaches are some nice foods to stock. They come with a very enjoyable natural sweetness, and when taken in moderation can help keep your blood sugar levels in check. Always keep in mind that when you make peaches part of your dessert like peach pie or peach cobbler, the glycemic index will change due to the other ingredients used. But when your peaches are eaten fresh, you have little to worry about as they do not spike up your blood sugar levels.

Pears

When trying to maintain a low blood sugar level, pears are some of the great fruits you can always choose. This delicious and nutritious fruit falls within the limit of low glycemic index fruits. They are mostly compared to apples but they differ from apples in that they bring a different mix of nutrients to the table. They equally differ in their unique flavor and grittier texture.

They will help you along with your daily fiber requirements. They make great side dishes and can be effectively incorporated into a number of recipes for main dishes. Always try to lay your hands on some organic pears that are in season, as they come with great taste and lacks the toxins the conventional pears come laden with.

Grapes

Most people believe grapes should be avoided whenever you are eating with keeping your blood sugar levels low in mind. But the fact that they are naturally sweet does not mean they come with an unhealthy or harmful glycemic index.

There are different types of grapes you can go for such as the red and the white grapes. The great thing about grapes that make them superfoods is the fact that they can be enjoyed directly as raw fruits. You can equally take a glass of organic grape juice once in a while and the glycemic index will still fall within the same range.

Milk

You can enjoy your delicious and nutritious glass of milk whenever you like without any fear of your blood sugar levels skyrocketing. Milk provides your body with adequate amount of calcium And vitamin D. Milk can be easily incorporated into a number of recipes and foods, so makes sure it is on your list of favorite superfoods if you want your blood sugar levels to remain low.

Yogurt

In recent years, yogurt have become more popular due to its links to digestive benefits. These digestive benefits that come from yogurts come as a result of their ability to provide the body with some good bacteria. Some yogurt brands even come with additional strains of digestive bacteria to provide additional support. Always go for brands that contain no kind of artificial sweeteners to keep your low blood sugar dreams alive. The all-natural and organic yogurt brands will always provide your body with good nutrients without spiking up your blood sugar levels.

Lentils

Lentils are getting more recommendations these days as a wonderful food to incorporate into your diet. It is one of those foods that are often overlooked when it comes to maintaining a low blood sugar conscious lifestyle. Experts recommend you eat lentils several times a week due to their ability to help you feel full for longer and keeping your blood sugar levels stable. Lentils are also known to be rich in fiber, vitamins and minerals which makes them quite beneficial to your overall health and wellness.

Sweet potatoes

Sweet potatoes have received more attention as very healthy food option. Most celebrity talk show hosts like Oprah and Dr OZ have given this superfood thumbs up as a very helpful dietary aid.

They first became popular when they started appearing in restaurants as white potato replacements, and they are indeed healthier in many regards. Opting for sweet potatoes have been found to be a healthier choice than baked or mashed potatoes. Sweet potatoes can be eaten as chips or boiled. They can be incorporated in popular dishes like rice, beans, and several other such daily cuisines.

Brown Rice

Brown rice is often presented as healthier alternatives to white rice in some restaurants. Brown rice is known to comes with a lower glycemic index than white rice and comes with more nutrients since they have not undergone the refining processes white rice get subjected to.

Studies have shown that the body utilizes white rice the same way it utilizes pure glucose, which makes white rice unhealthy for your blood sugar levels.

Peanuts

Peanuts can be enjoyed as your delicious everyday snack. They have very low glycemic index and help you reduce your hunger pang intervals. They have the ability to help you hang on till the next meal without feeling the hunger pangs much. They have the ability to stabilize your blood sugar levels helping you stay alert and clearheaded.

You can use peanuts as requested in some recipes and add peanut butter to your smoothie to give it more flavor and protein content. Peanuts are also known to be good sources of good fat.

Conclusion

These are the top 25 superfoods foe keeping your blood sugar levels stable, but they are not the only foods that help you achieve this health benefit. Other foods you can take to help you maintain a healthy blood sugar level include: cashew, strawberries, green beans, plums and prunes, oranges, etc.

The several health risks high blood sugar exposes you to, especially if you have a case of diabetes makes it an issue of life and death. Monitoring and caring for your blood sugar may be all you need to stay alive for longer.

Managing this health condition may seem a bit difficult, but the fact that there are several measures one can take to prevent, care and manage it makes it easier to be handled. The most important aspect of managing your blood sugar levels is in monitoring what goes into your system.

Following the list of healthy foods provided to help you keep your blood sugar in check is of urgent importance. Eating the right foods that do not spike up your blood sugar levels and avoiding foods that cause a rise in your blood sugar levels will help you stay in top health at all times.

As in many other diseases, prevention and proper care is often easier and more affordable than medical treatments and cure. Make sure you follow your blood sugar level monitoring tips and care plans to maintain a healthy and stable blood sugar levels at all times.